ALLEN PHOTOGRA

CARE OF
THE OLDER HORSE

CONTENTS

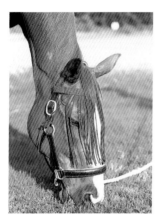

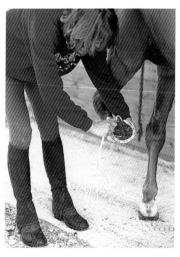

THE EFFECTS OF OLD AGE

Just as in humans, the ageing process is a gradual one, some horses will feel old at 12 years of age, while others are fine at the age of 20, or even older. As horses age they seem to have less resistance to cold weather, worms, viruses and skin diseases. Older horses need to be fed and looked after carefully if they are to continue working happily or to enjoy a healthy and contented retirement.

Depending on the type of life they have led and how quickly they have aged, some old horses are kept in retirement while others are still in full work. Many old horses are in semi-retirement, hacking out at weekends or being kept busy during the summer holidays. We start by looking at a year in the life of the older horse and examining the problems posed by the changing seasons of the year for both the working and retired horse.

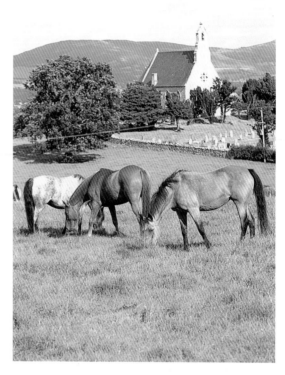

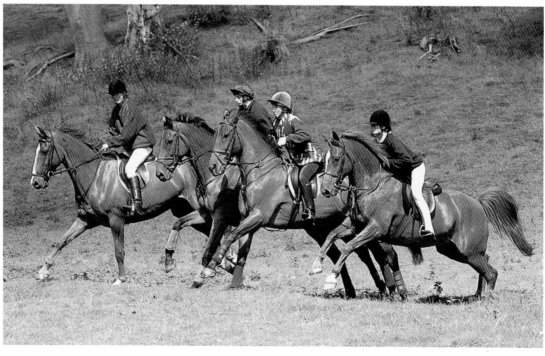

SPRING

After the long winter we will look forward to the spring but spring brings its own problems for the old or retired horse.

TOO MUCH GRASS

Nature intended the horse to get fat in the summer when grass is plentiful and thin in the winter when the grazing is sparse. Older horses that have wintered well and are only in light work or are retired, are likely to get too fat when the spring grass comes through. Any obese horse is at risk from laminitis, so it is very important to manage your grazing to prevent the horse getting fat. The paddock can be divided into smaller areas using electric fencing. The horse should only be allowed sufficient grazing to keep his condition without putting on weight. The rest of the field can be cut for hay or grazed by other horses which are less likely to get fat. Once the summer comes and the grass stops growing so quickly the horse can probably graze the whole area.

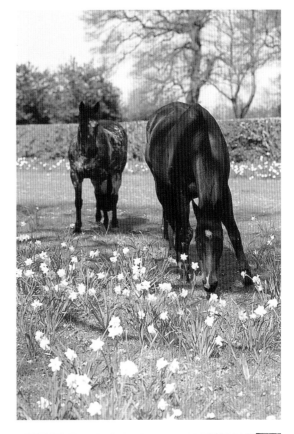

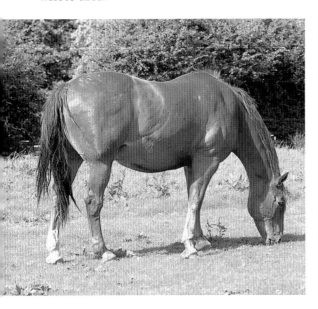

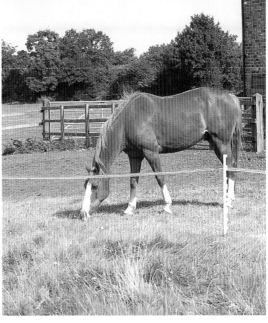

SUMMER

Although a pleasure for us, the summer can be a nightmare for horses out at grass: pestered by flies, short of grazing and exposed to the glare of the sun.

THE FLY PROBLEM

Horses and ponies at grass must be protected from fly nuisance; flies irritate horses causing runny eyes and possible injury as horses kick and stamp to get rid of the flies. Many thin-skinned horses lose condition, constantly keeping on the move to avoid the flies rather than grazing. Relief can be given by providing shelter, a fly fringe, a fly hood or treating the horse with a long-acting fly repellent. Many horses thrive best by being turned out at night and brought into the stable during the heat of the day.

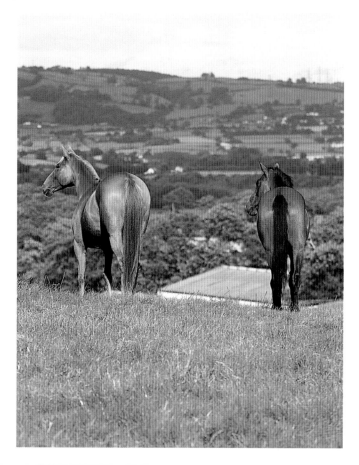

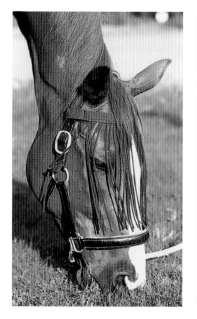

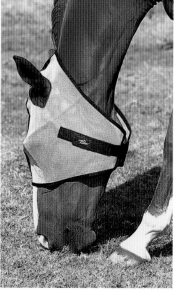

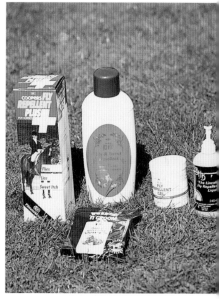

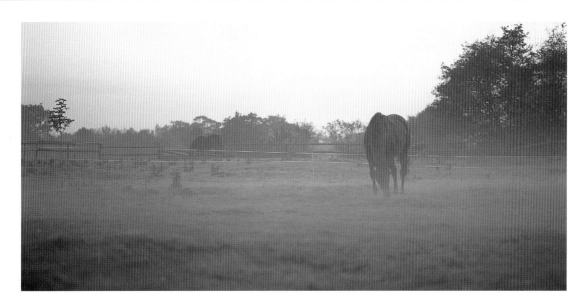

TOO LITTLE GRASS

Hot, dry summers can leave horses at grass with very little to eat. It may be necessary to supplement the older horse's diet with hay to make up for the shortage of grazing. If the horse is still losing condition he will need to be given concentrate feed as well. It is also essential to keep a close eye on the water supply as horses drink more in hot weather. If water is provided in buckets, rather than in a self-filling trough you will need to check the water twice a day. A retired horse takes nearly as much looking after as a working horse; just because you are not riding him does not mean you can get away with not checking the horse, the field, the fencing and the water every day.

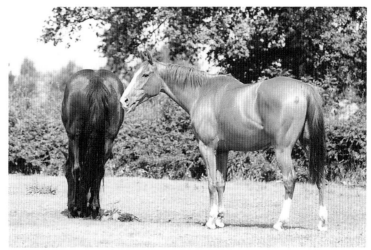

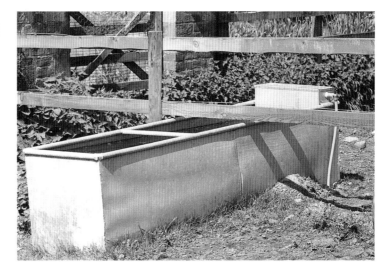

WINTER

The winter can be a vulnerable time for the retired horse. Many thoroughbred-type horses will not thrive wintered out. Before retiring this sort of horse you must consider the quality of life they will lead when they are retired. They will probably have to be stabled at night during the winter and will cost as much in time and money as a working horse.

RUGS

To rug or not to rug? Most ponies and part-bred horses will grow a thick winter coat that will protect them from all but the worst weather. The shape of the horse and the way the mane, tail and feathers grow is designed to keep the vulnerable parts of their bodies dry. Horses that are kept out during the winter should not have their manes and tails pulled or their feathers trimmed.

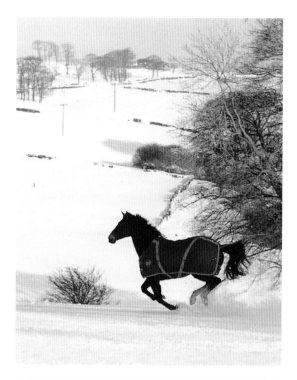

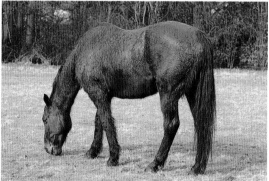

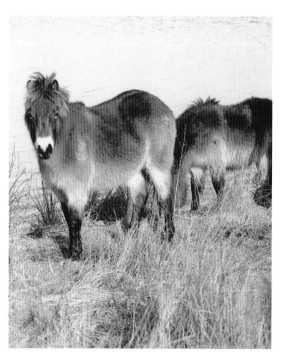

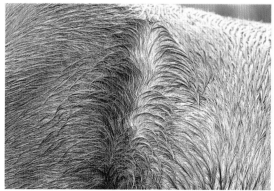

Thoroughbreds and fine ponies may need to be rugged to stop them getting cold and wet and losing condition. There are many types of material and many styles of turn-out rug but the most important thing is that the rug fits. Too often the rug slips back or sideways and cuts into the horse's withers. If a horse is wearing a badly fitting rug for 24 hours a day, he will soon be rubbed raw. It is better to have no rug than an ill-fitting one.

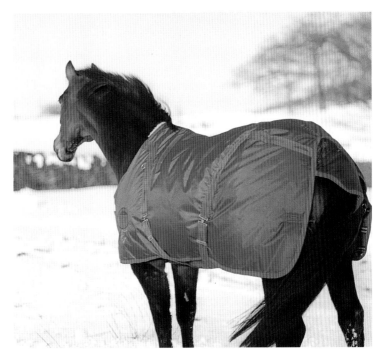

SHELTER

The out-wintered horse must be able to find shelter from the wind and rain. It is particularly important that the area where the hay is fed is sheltered as this is where the horse will spend a lot of time. Shelter can be provided by a purpose-built shelter, a stout high hedge or the lee of a hill.

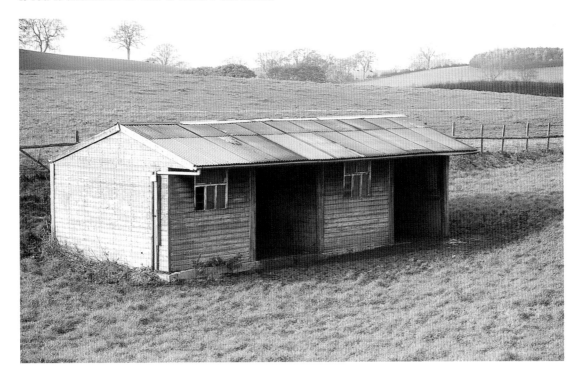

FIELD CARE

Inevitably as the winter progresses the horse's feet will churn up or 'poach' the field. Unshod feet do far less damage than shod ones, so the retired horse should have his shoes removed and the feet trimmed regularly. If your fields are wet and do not drain well the horse may have to come in during the wetter months, usually after Christmas until the spring. Again this should be considered before making the decision to retire the horse.

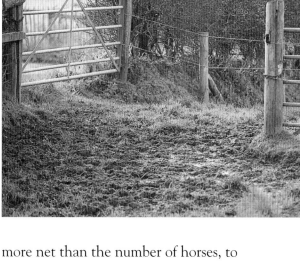

FEEDING AT GRASS

Nearly all old, retired horses living out during the winter will need extra feed, especially during cold, wet spells of weather. As the quantity and quality of the grazing falls in the autumn, the horse should be fed hay before he starts to lose condition. Hay can be fed in nets, hay racks or on the ground. Hay nets should be hung sufficiently high so that the horse cannot catch a foot in an empty net and there should be one more net than the number of horses, to avoid squabbling. Hay racks should be designed so that the horse cannot catch himself on any sharp edges or bang his head. Feeding hay on the ground is wasteful but quick and easy. If there are several horses in the field the piles of hay should be placed well apart with one more pile than there are horses, otherwise one bully can hog the whole lot!

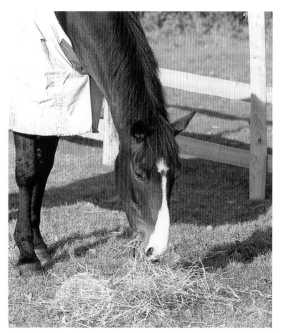

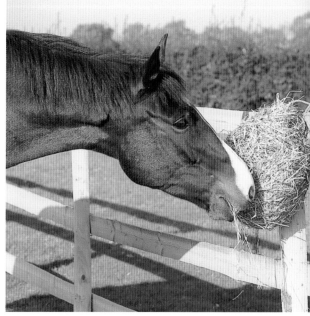

STABLING

The old horse who is still in work is likely to need stabling at night. The amount of work the horse is doing and the thickness of his coat will determine what sort of clip he should have and how many rugs he will need. A useful clip for the horse in light work is a belly clip where only the hair on the belly and the underside of the neck is removed.

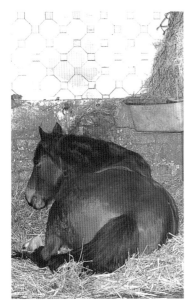
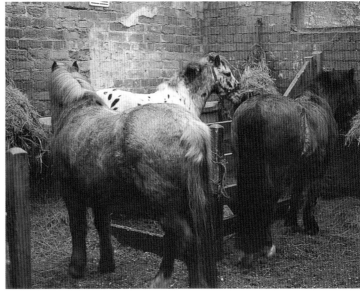

COMPANIONSHIP

Horses are social animals and the retiree will appreciate having a friend to share his retirement all year round.

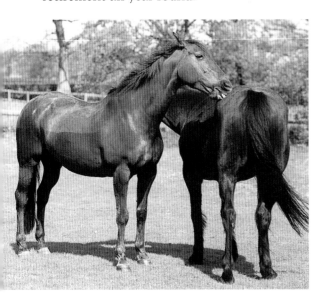
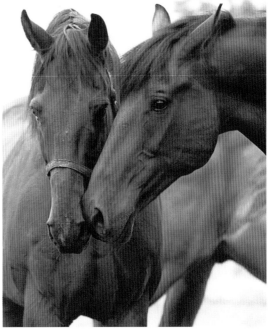

ROUTINE CARE

The older horse will still need regular attention. If he is kept at grass but is still in light work he will need to be cleaned before he is ridden. The mud can be knocked off using a dandy brush but he should not be given a thorough groom with a body brush as this will remove the protective grease from his coat. Particular attention should be paid to the legs, checking for signs of cracked heels and mud fever. Even the retired horse will need his eyes, nose, dock and feet regularly inspected and cleaned. Runny eyes can be sponged with water or cold tea, indeed the used tea bag makes a useful disposable wipe.

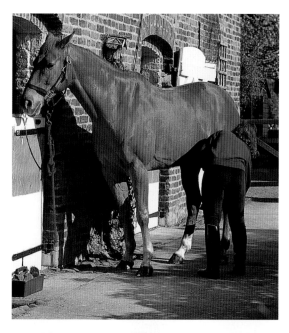

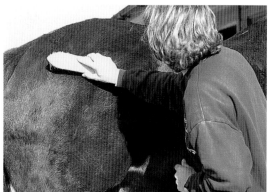

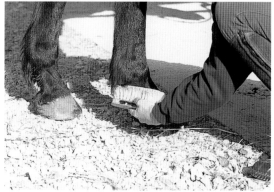

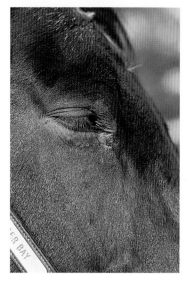

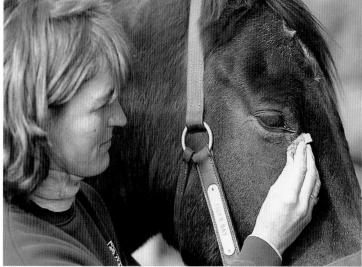

Separate sponges or cloths should be kept for wiping the horse's nose and cleaning under his dock. The shod horse should have his feet picked out daily and the shoes checked for signs that they need replacing. The unshod horse should have his feet trimmed regularly by the farrier. There should be a regular and effective worming programme for the older horse. The timing and frequency of worming will depend on the number of horses in the field and how 'horse sick' the pasture is. Generally the horse will have to be wormed every 6–10 weeks throughout the whole year. Once the horse is retired you may decide that he no longer needs an annual 'flu jab, however it is essential that his vaccinations against tetanus are kept up to date.

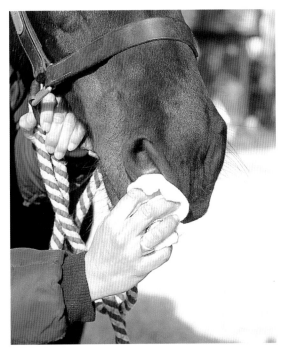

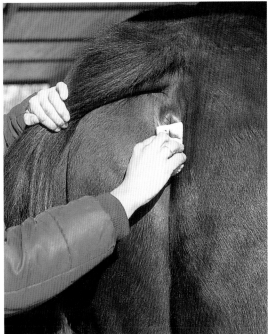

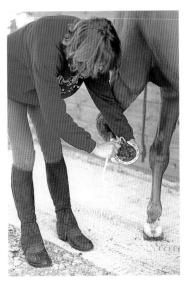

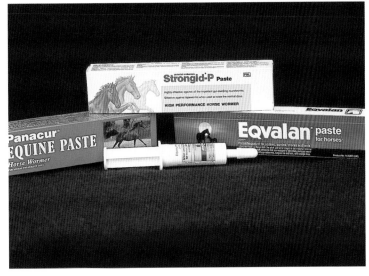

WORKING THE OLDER HORSE

Old horses can lead an active life until well into their 20s; in recognition of this there are show classes specially for veteran horses. Many horses have competed at the highest level into their late teens and then 'retired'

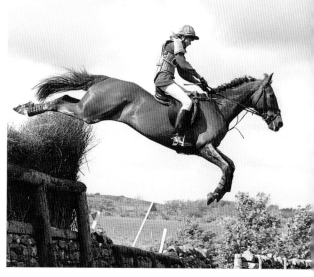

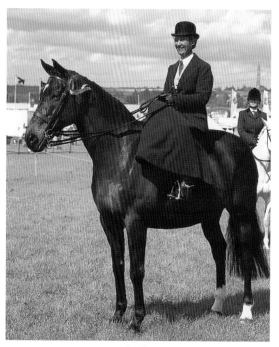

to the hunting field. Horses are active creatures; many that have been accustomed to a competition regime are happier kept in work than being turned out in the field where they feel bored and neglected. Indeed, these horses often make excellent schoolmasters for young riders or in riding schools and colleges.

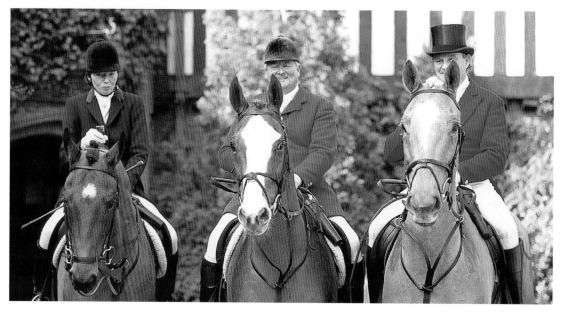

It is a mistake to give the older horse far less work to 'preserve' him for his work. He probably needs to be even more fit and well than his younger counterpart to cope with demanding work such as hunting or competing. Remember, he does not have the resilience of youth. It is worth considering the following points.

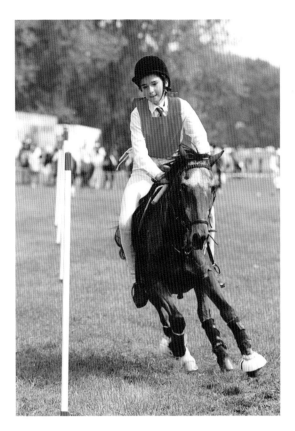

- Do not let him get fat and unfit during the summer when there is lots of grass, keep him 'ticking over' by riding him two or three times a week. It is highly stressful on joints, tendons, ligaments and muscles to be allowed to get soft and then be subjected to an intense training programme to return to fitness.

- Do not give the old horse long days, be it competing or hunting.

- Do not keep him standing in the horsebox for hours, he will stiffen up and the hours a horse spends out of the stable are nearly as tiring as the hours he spends under saddle.

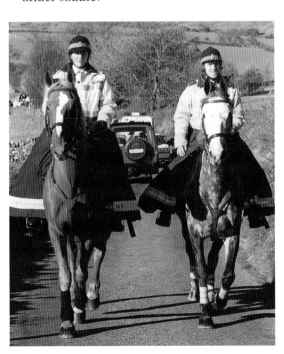

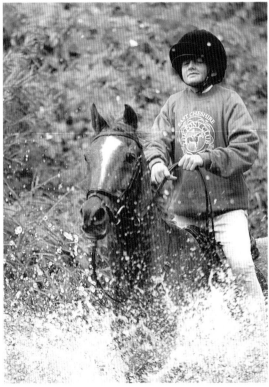

FEEDING

Just because your horse has reached his fifteenth or sixteenth birthday does not mean that you have to change his feed. Let your eye and the horse's condition and performance tell you when, or indeed if, you need to alter his diet. Telltale signs include:

- dropping condition during the winter;
- losing condition in the summer when the grazing is sparse, even if he is being fed hay;
- lacking energy;
- losing his top line, i.e. the muscles of the neck, back and hindquarters.

SPECIAL REQUIREMENTS

Many old horses have lost some of their teeth or have sharp teeth, this reduces their ability to chew hay, grains and cubes. Pain and discomfort from arthritis may stop the horse moving around and grazing freely, as well as possibly reducing his appetite. As horses age, their digestive efficiency decreases and they need more energy for everyday life. Older horses also need higher levels of good quality protein as well as higher levels of calcium and phosphorus in their rations.

VETERAN DIETS

To help him keep his condition the older horse's diet needs to be:

- very tasty;
- easy to eat;
- rich in nutrients.

Most feed manufacturers make mixes specially for veteran horses and ponies which are rich in energy and protein and contain higher levels of minerals and vitamins.

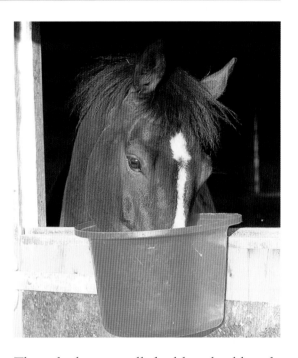

These feeds are usually highly palatable soft mixes which are easy to eat. The majority of manufacturers design their range of feeds to be compatible with each other; veteran or conditioning feed may make up all or just part of your concentrate ration, depending on the horse's individual requirements. If you are in any doubt, ring the company and ask their nutritionist to help you sort out your horse's diet.

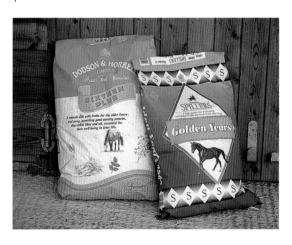

FORMULATING YOUR OWN RATIONS

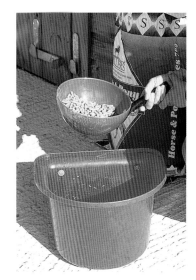

If your horse has difficulty chewing, try soaking cubes to
make a sort of soup, or try feeding boiled barley, soaked
sugar beet pulp, Alfa Beet or soaked alfalfa pellets. Hay can
be made easier to eat by damping it. If the old horse's teeth
are so bad that he cannot eat hay, crushed high fibre cubes,
chopped hay or chaff can be fed to provide bulk. Horses
that cannot graze effectively can have fresh grass cut daily
for them during the summer. While a compound feed will
be formulated to meet all your horse's needs, these 'straight'
feeds must be balanced by using a broad spectrum mineral
and vitamin supplement. All horses appreciate succulents
such as carrots and apples, these should be sliced length-
ways so that they cannot get stuck in the horse's throat
causing choke. During cold weather, old horses will need more feed: boiled barley is appetis-
ing and easy to eat while sunflower or soya oil provides non-heating, concentrated energy.

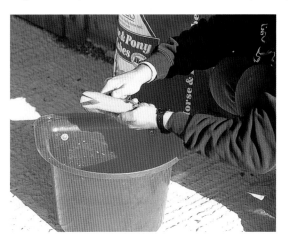
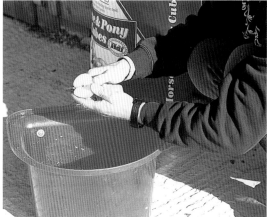

HOW MUCH TO FEED

The amount of feed your horse or pony
needs to eat will depend on a number of
factors.

- Size – smaller animals need less.
- Condition – lean horses will need more
  to eat than those in good condition.
  However, as older horses can be more
  prone to digestive upsets, do not be
  tempted to overfeed them. Putting condition on a horse can be a slow process. It is
  important to assess the horse's condition

and the quantity and quality of the grazing every week.
- Work – as with all horses, the older horse
  will need more feed than the resting
  horse.
- Time of year – as the weather gets colder
  more feed is often needed to help the
  horse maintain his condition.
- A hot summer may mean sparse grazing in
  which case more feed might be needed.
- Look after the horse's teeth and feet and
  have an effective worming programme.

AILMENTS

If he is to stay happy and healthy the old horse needs special attention. As horses age they become more susceptible to problems such as arthritis and cataracts. The retired horse who is out at grass all year round may be prey to laminitis, mud fever and rain scald.

ARTHRITIS

Old horses are often stiff after a hard day's work, this is often caused by arthritis. Arthritis is a disease of the joints; in older horses, wear and tear may lead to cartilage within the joint breaking down and being replaced by bone. The joints of the fetlock and hock are most commonly affected. While there are anti-inflammatory drugs that the vet can prescribe, there are natural alternatives to these drugs. Old favourites are cod liver oil and cider vinegar. Supplements based on cod liver oil and containing essential fatty acids have been specially developed for horses and claim to be able to

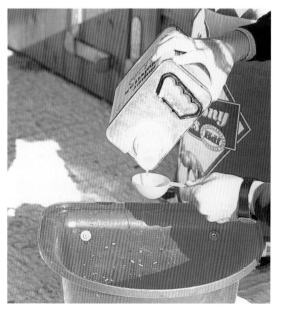

relieve the pain and stiffness associated with arthritis and rheumatism.

More recently on the market is a substance called MSM (methylsulphonylmethane), a natural anti-inflammatory, which has been claimed to have had significant results in arthritic humans and dogs as well as horses. It is said to reduce inflammation and promote blood circulation thus alleviating pain and helping the body heal itself.

One thing is certain, you must take action to preserve your horse and prolong his active life *before* the signs of wear and tear become apparent. Once a horse is persistently unsound, even if only mildly, stable management and feeding are unlikely to have much effect.

TEETH

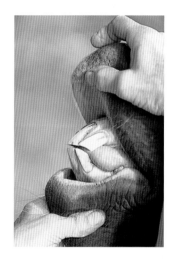

From the age of five the horse has a full set of adult permanent teeth. Up until the age of 12 the teeth grow continuously to compensate for the constant wear they receive grinding the horse's fibrous diet. After this the teeth are gradually worn down and eventually old horses will lose their teeth. As the teeth wear out the horse may experience difficulty eating and the diet will have to be adjusted accordingly. All horses, even when retired, should have their teeth checked twice a year and rasped if necessary. This can be done by the vet or horse dentist.

PITUITARY CANCER (CUSHING'S DISEASE)

The pituitary gland is found just under the horse's brain, its role is to control the endocrine system thus being responsible for the general metabolism of the horse. Older horses can develop a benign cancer of the pituitary gland which results in them losing condition, drinking a lot and possibly becoming diabetic. One of the first signs you may see is that the horse fails to lose his winter coat. These horses are prone to developing laminitis and should be carefully managed; they need a high fibre, low sugar ration and a close eye should be kept on their condition.

LAMINITIS

Laminitis is a problem usually associated with fat ponies who have eaten too much rich spring grass but, it must be remembered, horses are equally susceptible to this problem. The result of laminitis is a disruption of the blood supply to the foot which causes pain. In severe or neglected cases the pedal bone within the foot rotates and the animal is said to 'founder'. With prompt veterinary attention this can be

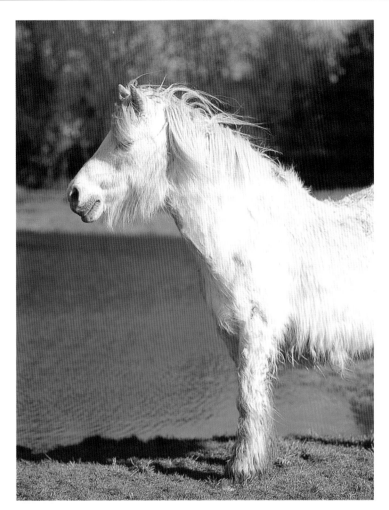

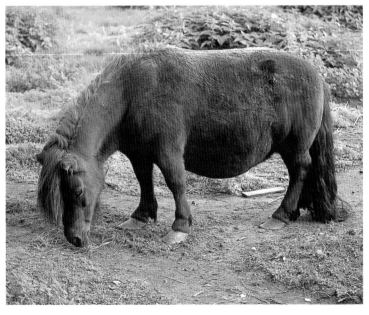

avoided and a full recovery can be made. The recovering patient should be fed a maintenance ration based on good quality hay but the animal's access to grass should be strictly limited. However, the animal must not be starved, this can result in a condition called hyperlipaemia, which is potentially fatal. Remember most older horses and ponies do not need a lot of concentrate feed unless they lack condition or are working hard. Any concentrate ration fed should be based on digestible fibre, perhaps including alfalfa chaff, unmolassed sugar beet pulp and high fibre horse and pony cubes. A suitable supplement, perhaps one that encourages hoof growth and horn quality, can also be included. It may also be useful to feed a probiotic to try to keep the bacterial conditions within the horse's gut as stable as possible. High starch and high sugar feeds must be avoided. If the horse needs more energy or condition, oil can be added.

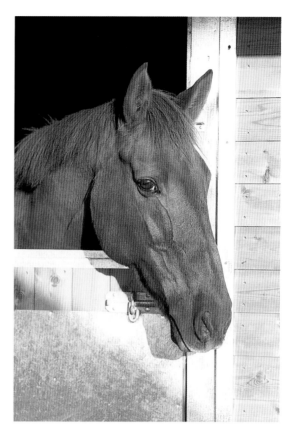

Any overweight horse or pony is susceptible to laminitis, this puts retired horses that are 'good-doers' in the high-risk category and they should be managed in a similar way to any pony that has had laminitis. Access to pasture must be limited and their body weight strictly controlled. Great care must be taken to be aware of any changes in the grass growth, for example if it rains after a dry spell in the summer the horse should be stabled and only allowed to graze for a short time every day.

MUD FEVER AND RAIN SCALD

Mud fever and rain scald are skin problems that affect horses and ponies living in wet and muddy conditions. Constant wetting of the skin allows infection by a bug called *Dermotophilus congolensis*, resulting in sore scabby areas. The condition is called mud fever if the legs are affected and rain scald if the neck, back and hindquarters are affected. If there is mud fever on the lower leg, there can be considerable swelling and the horse is often lame. The first step in

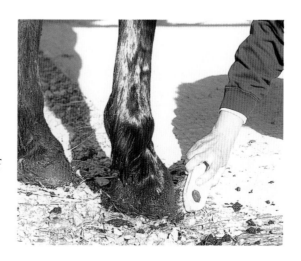

treating mud fever is to stable the horse to keep the skin dry. The next step is to remove the scabs and dress the skin with a soothing antibiotic ointment. In severe cases the scabs become infected and the vet should be called as the horse will need a course of antibiotics. Horses that are prone to rain scald should wear a New Zealand rug and have access to a field shelter. It is more difficult to prevent mud fever; the horse's legs should be carefully examined every day during the winter for signs of cracked heels, soreness and scabs. When the fields become wet it may be necessary to wash off the mud, dry the legs and apply petroleum jelly or zinc and castor oil cream to the heels and pasterns to help waterproof the legs and prevent the problem.

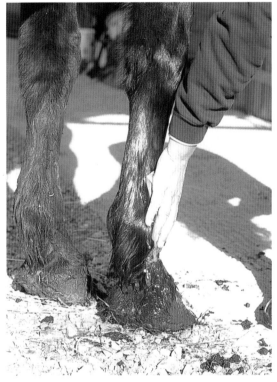

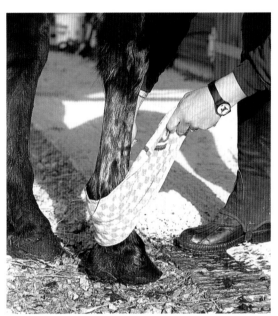

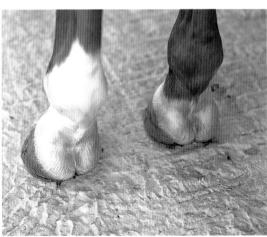

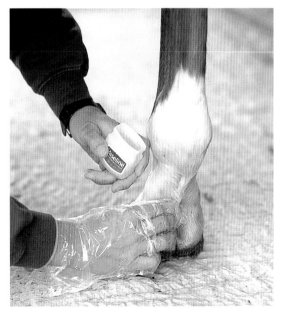

CATARACTS

Older horses may develop cataracts, a condition where the lens of the eye becomes cloudy. Sometimes cataracts do not affect the horse's sight but progressive cataracts can eventually lead to blindness. If the horse's sight is affected you may notice him stumbling, shying or bumping into things. The vet can diagnose the problem by examining the eye with an opthalmascope. This horse's eye has been injured leading to its cloudy appearance.

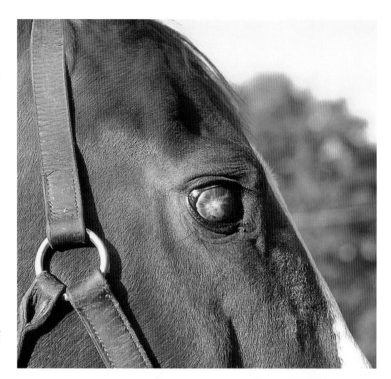

LACK OF CONDITION

Older horses may not keep their condition as well as they did in their youth, especially if they are still in work. Feeding greater quantities of corn may merely result in over exuberance and you hitting the deck! The best option is to try to feed the horse in a way which helps the horse help himself by enhancing digestive efficiency. Try feeding a mix specially formulated for veteran horses. If the horse still lacks condition, add a probiotic or yeast supplement to the feed, these act to stabilise the conditions within the gut and help the horse get the most out of his food.

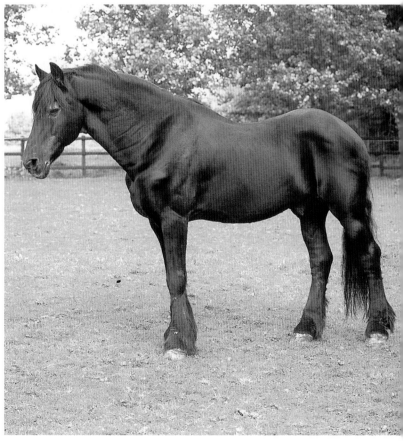

OBESITY

Fat horses are more prone to laminitis and more strain is put on the body systems. Even if retired, the overweight horse needs to get slimmer. Just as with humans there is no easy way to get slim, the horse must simply go on a diet and get more, controlled exercise if he is to lose weight. For the best long-term results the horse's weight loss should be gradual, accomplished by a combination of a lower energy diet and more work. The protein, fibre, mineral and vitamin levels of the diet should be kept at maintenance levels while the energy is gradually reduced so that the horse burns up body fat to provide the energy needed. With the stabled horse, the first thing to do is to cut the concentrate feed to a minimum. The next step is to reduce the hay ration. The horse should be kept on a non-edible bedding and his hay fed in a net with small holes so that it takes longer to eat. Feeding good quality oat or barley straw can be a useful way of providing the fat horse with bulk and fibre without oversupplying energy. Straw is eaten slowly and needs a

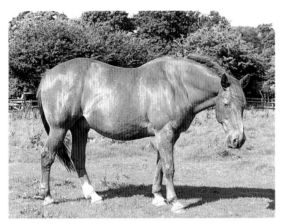

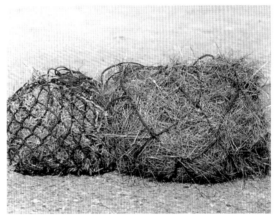

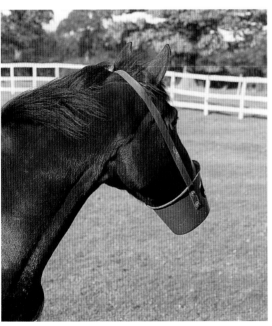

great deal of chewing thus keeping the horse occupied and helping to prevent the dieting horse getting bored. If the horse is at grass the grazing will have to be restricted, perhaps to only an hour morning and evening. He will have to spend the rest of the time stabled or confined to a bare 'starvation' paddock. The horse should get a mineral or vitamin supplement mixed in a handful of chaff to ensure that he remains healthy during weight loss. It is possible to buy muzzles which allow the horse to bite only tiny amounts of grass at a time. This keeps the horse occupied and working hard for each mouthful. A muzzle is also a useful way of stopping ponies getting too fat in the spring.

THE FINAL DECISION

One of the most painful and distressing decisions that any animal owner ever has to make is when to have the animal put down. Very few horses or ponies die naturally of old age which means that it is a problem that the owner of an old horse or pony is going to have to face sooner or later. There is no easy way to make the decision but most vets will be very helpful and give you an objective assessment of your horse's health, condition and quality of life. You will know in your heart of hearts when the time has come and for your own peace of mind you need to make the decision at the right time. Remember you owe it to your horse to let him end his life with dignity.

Some owners find a second opinion from an uninvolved party helpful to confirm that the correct decision has been made. If the horse is insured, the insurance company must be notified as their permission is needed before the horse is put down in all but emergency cases.

You can plan the timing, for example if your vet advises you that it would not be fair or kind to put the horse through another winter, you may decide to let the horse have one last summer at grass. You must, however, also bear in mind that some horses find the heat and flies of summer harder to tolerate than the cold of winter.

If the horse is fit to travel and free from

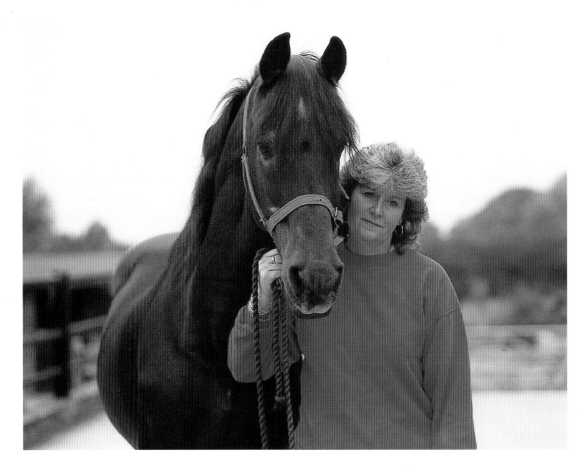

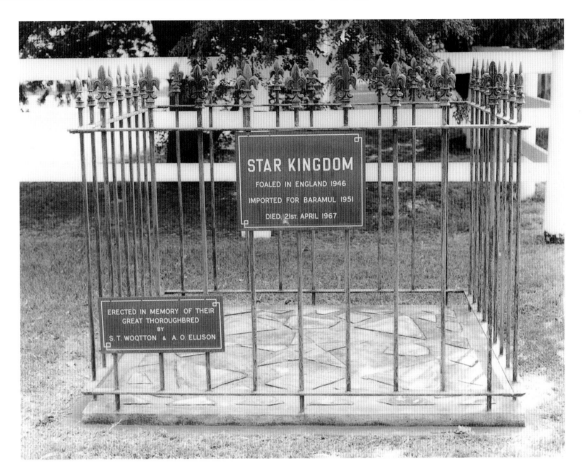

STAR KINGDOM

FOALED IN ENGLAND 1946

IMPORTED FOR BARAMUL 1951

DIED 21st APRIL 1967

ERECTED IN MEMORY OF THEIR
GREAT THOROUGHBRED
BY
S. T. WOOTTON & A. O. ELLISON

medication, he can be taken to an approved horse abattoir and full carcass value can be obtained. An appointment can be made and there will be veterinary supervision. Alternatively the horse can be taken to the vet, the local hunt kennels or the knacker's yard. These professional people will carry out the task efficiently and compassionately.

Some owners have their horse put down at home by the vet. He will use a gun, captive bolt pistol or intravenous injection. The horse is usually sedated before being given a fatal injection and if the horse has a fear of vets and needles this can prolong the procedure. If the horse is destroyed at home the body will have to be disposed of: burial requires National Rivers Authority permission. Some horse abattoirs offer a cremation service for these horses which, while expensive, offers many owners peace of mind.

You may wish to be with your horse during his last moments but do realise that it will be a traumatic experience and it may be better to let the professionals get on with the job without having to worry about you as well.

Above all, remember the need to put the horse's welfare before your own sentiment.

ACKNOWLEDGEMENTS

I would like to thank Joanna Prestwich and her, sometimes reluctant, equine models for all the photographs. Also, Chelford Horse & Country, Knutsford Road, Chelford, Cheshire SK1 9AS, for providing materials for use in the photographs.

British Library Cataloguing-in-Publication Data.
A catalogue record for this book is available from the
British Library

ISBN 0.85131.734.0

Published in Great Britain in 1999 by
J. A. Allen & Company Limited,
1 Lower Grosvenor Place, Buckingham Palace Road,
London, SW1W OEL

Design and Typesetting by Paul Saunders
Series editor Jane Lake
Colour Separation by Tenon & Polert Colour Scanning Ltd.
Printed in Hong Kong by Dah Hua Printing Press Co. Ltd.